Weight Loss Foods Mistakes

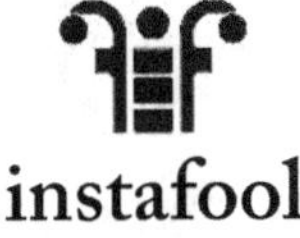

instafool

Presents

Weight Loss Foods Mistakes

15 Healthy Foods to Avoid when Losing Weight and Dieting

Instafo

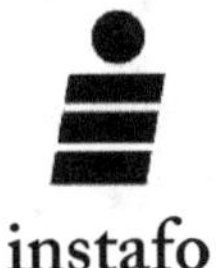

instafo

While attempts have been made to verify the information contained within this publication, neither the author nor the publisher assumes any responsibility for errors, omissions, interpretation or usage of the subject matter herein.

This publication contains the opinions and ideas of its author and is intended for informational purpose only. The author and publisher shall in no event be held liable for any loss or other damages incurred from the usage of this publication.

*Note this is not intended to substitute any medical advice. Always consult with a physician or a professional in matters related to your health.

ISBN 978-1-687-47154-3

Printed in the United States of America

First Edition

FOOL'S GUIDE

PROLOGUE:
The Fool Card

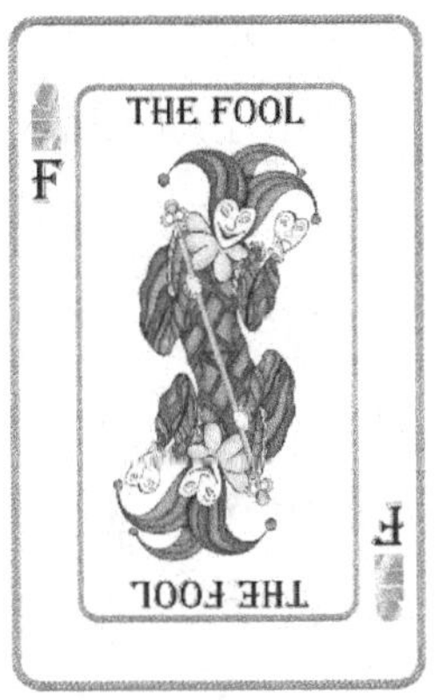

"A fool thinks himself to be wise, but a wise man knows himself to be a fool." – **William Shakespeare**

Ready to have your fortune read? Then pick a card...any card. Ah, congratulations! You have selected the **Fool card.** *Don't* *despair!* It is the most powerful one, being the omnipotent wild card as well as the first card in a tarot deck with the number 0, that represents new journey and new solution available with unlimited optimism, unexhausted enthusiasm, and undiscovered opportunities, because to a fool...anything is possible!

Yet, the fool is "nobody's fool" but is *secretly* the wisest of all, able to pull strings in the most dire situations due to a sharp wit, astute acumen, erudite knowledge, diligent resourcefulness, and perceptive observation of the world and what goes on around. Indeed cunning, evasive, and elusive to get ahead without being ensnared by the same established rules others played by, the fool is able to think and see things outside of the box.

With that said, you can learn a lot from the fool through all their intentional and unintentional antics.

Nobody likes to hear the truth. *The truth hurts...but is honest.* Historically, only the fool was sly enough to get away with the most unfavorable truth in the royal court from knowing everything that went on, without getting his own head chopped and served on a king's silver platter for the hidden genius disguised as superficial foolishness. Perhaps a forgivable trickster in this regard, the fool was, nonetheless and above all, a true survival of the fittest and a formidable force to behold.

If you want to possess the great wisdom of the fool in a modern era of instant information, look no further because you have found your tarot calling card: **Instafool.**

Being an Instafool is for those fools who dare question and go up against conventional knowledge, by exploring the polar opposite side of the coin which nobody else is willing do and by exposing the cold-hard truth which nobody else is willing to admit, in order to gain better perspective, bigger picture, and wider spectrum covering all aspects of everything in any area.

While the fool may be a joker, the Instafool is no joke or laughing matter. Being the Instafool is about being a renaissance visionary trailblazing innovative ideas and being an inquisitive intellect uncovering controversial truths and unapologetically and shamelessly willing to educate those truths, even when gaining ridicules from others.

It's better to be an Instafool than be fooled in a world full of so much instant MISinformation. *Know thy truth by knowing thy untruth.* That's the key role of the Instafool.

This now sums up the Instafool and your tarot card reading. What shall you do now is entirely up to you...

Shall you be audacious enough to follow this path of an Instafool?

ANECDOTE:
The Fool Iffy

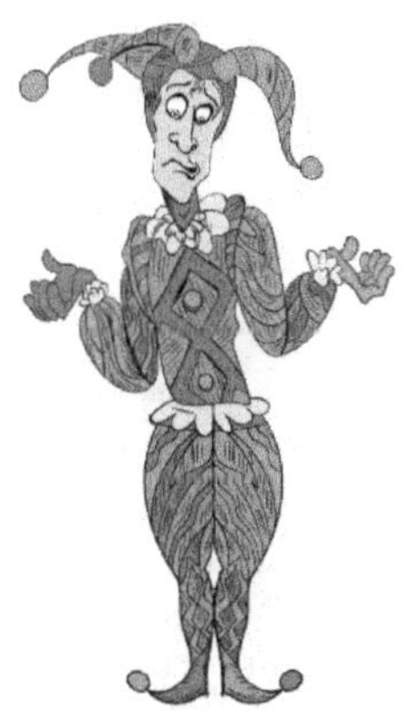

Meet "Iffy the Fool" of the high king. He's the fool for the royal court's amusement by entertaining them, but more importantly...indirectly educating them with his endless clumsy antics at the expense of his competence and confidence...for all to see what not do and avoid.

Don't be like Iffy the Fool. Be the opposite of him through learning from his mistakes and doing the opposite of what he does.

Whether intentional or unintentional, the wise fool in disguised accidentally becomes the best teacher around.

He shall now be your guide...

F(OOL) ACT AT PLAY: Surprisingly Unhealthy Healthy Foods

Want to lose weight? You are not alone. Millions of people would love to drop a few (or many!) pounds, but they struggle to succeed. They would hit the gym with all the fiery motivation that would make the sun burn bright for the next millennium without getting the desired result.

The missing factor? It should come as of no surprise that getting in peak shape is more than about working out but also watching what you eat to achieve weight loss.

However—what hardly anybody ever talks about—it's just as important (if not more) to watch what you should _NOT_ eat, especially those supposedly "healthy foods."

When people want to trim down, most of the time they are aware that when they go grocery shopping, they should select fruits, vegetables, and other healthy (low-fat or nutrient-dense) foods. But with so many options on the shelves, people may be tempted to grab items like low-fat yogurt, low-fat milk, and things that seem healthy, like (first spoiler alert) cereal. After all, while growing up, we were told that eating cereal in the morning was good for us.

You're probably thinking that there's nothing wrong with the foods we mentioned above. But the truth is that there are actually several risks that come with eating certain foods when trying to **"lose weight"** and keep it off forever.

You have to remember that losing weight is about adopting new routines and a new lifestyle that comes with, perhaps, eating smaller portions. And you need to know what really is—or is not—good for you without having to think about it. Losing weight also comes with a culture. In other words, you should have a certain relationship with food so you know what to avoid (like, perhaps, pork or processed food).

Information is key. So, getting just enough information before deciding what to eat when you are on a diet can make a big difference. With the right information, you will realize that not all traditionally healthy and "low-cal" foods are good for you when it comes to maintaining a healthy weight.

Here's why some of the commonly-believed healthy foods may do more harm than good:

- They are packed with sugar, syrup, and other addictives; this is especially true with many weight loss meals that are labeled as low-fat. There are going to be some trade-offs in order to be marketed as healthy.

- They might make you hungrier, which doesn't help curb your cravings. That's what happens with sugary foods because they taste good but often lack actual nutritional consistency.

- They provide no energy if you are also exercising to lose weight. You have to remember that your body should be able to sustain a certain endurance while working out (no blackouts or pain in the joints), so packing it with enough water and nutrient-dense food is always a must.

- They can be harmful in the long run and contribute to obesity or a high sugar level in the blood. This is a major trap because by believing certain foods are healthy, you rely excessively on them thinking that you're getting the benefit, while the revere effect is unknowingly in play.

Getting to know what you really put on your plate, especially when it comes to weight loss, is the same thing as when you wipe your airplane seat and tray table with sanitary wipes for precautionary reasons. This will allow you to be more careful and more successful at not exposing yourself to failure or other problems.

<u>Note</u>: Before moving on, we just want to put out there that we are not blasting these subsequent foods as completely unhealthy; they're just not ideal when it comes to your <u>goal</u> of *losing weight*. In any other case scenario, they're fine as part of a healthy balanced nutritional diet.

<u>TASK</u>: Time to do a small "cleaning up the pantry and fridge" task. First, move all the natural and generally labeled "healthy" foods in your pantry and fridge to the right side (for the time being). As you continue going through our list of foods to avoid, move those healthy foods that are potentially harmful to your weight loss program from the right side to the left side. This includes foods like healthy meals bought from your nearest grocery store, as well as some yogurts, cereal, etc.

Let's now jump into our first healthy food to avoid.

MISTAKE #1:
Misleading "Low-Fat" and "Fat-Free" Labels

Don't let those healthy-sounding labels fool you. From now on, try to stay away from anything with labels such as "low-fat" or "fat-free." Even if the food resembles or tastes like what your mother cooks for you when you are visiting, or even if it's advertised on TV, steer clear from it.

<u>REASONS</u>: They are filled with preservatives—sometimes *a lot of sugar*—to add taste. So if these foods are part of your regular weekly meals then your weight loss program might be doomed from the start. This is confirmed by Marion Nestle, a professor of nutrition, food studies, and public health at New York University. She said the food industry

substitutes vegetable fats for animal fats in such great proportions that when it comes to low-fat and fat-free meals, they end up having the same calorie content as regular versions of these meals.

<u>BENCHMARK</u>: Stay away from sugars and harmful preservatives by cooking your own meals a day in advance. Or if you are a very busy person, cook five-course meals and store them in your fridge and freezer for easy re-heating another day. Learning how to make your own yogurts, healthy pasta, etc., at home is also beneficial.

<u>BENEFITS</u>: By making your own meals, you know exactly what you are putting into them and what winds up in your body. That way, you'll know if you will be able to burn all those calories later on. When you see foods labeled "low-fat" and "fat-free" in the store, it's comparable to someone selling fake jewelry but advertising it as real. You are tricked into buying the jewelry, then you realize later when it starts to fade that it was not real gold or silver after all. The promise of "low-fat" and "fat-free" foods (at least most

of them) is the same. You think they will help you lose weight. But they won't. You'll be indirectly putting on the pounds.

<u>TASK</u>: As a small task, start getting rid of all the "low-fat" and "fat-free" foods from your home. An easy way to know which foods to get rid of is to think of all the sweet-tasting "low-fat" and "fat-free" foods like yogurt, cream, coffee creamer, ice cream, etc. Move them to the left side of your fridge or pantry (as a continuation of your previous task). Then once you have identified and moved everything, get rid of everything that's on the left side. Of course, we don't want you to waste food. Consider giving these items to the food banks or needy and people who don't need to lose weight.

MISTAKE #2:
Secretly Fattening Salads

Pre-made salads sure are convenient, aren't they? They are especially easy when you are in a hurry or need to eat lunch on the go. And if it's a salad, it must be healthy, right? *Not necessarily!*

What's the kicker? Salads are not limited to lettuce (or other lettuce supplements) and a few other vegetables. Overall, you can fill your tummy with a healthy and well-balanced salad. But eating pre-made salads regularly can lead to weight gain and sabotage your weight loss plan, preventing you from getting the results you want.

<u>REASONS</u>: The problem is not so much with the lettuce, tomatoes, and chicken they put in your salad. It is mostly the high-calorie dressings or all the other unhealthy ingredients like cheddar cheese and bacon that they often put in pre-made salads at the store or from fast-food restaurants. Kathy MacManus, director of the Department of Nutrition at Brigham and Women's Hospital in Boston, warns that dressings used for pre-made salads usually add a lot of calories, sodium, and sugar.

<u>BENCHMARK</u>: Learn to make your own healthy and delicious salads, and pick the right condiments to add to it. You should also learn to make your own salad dressing, which is not as complicated as you may think. The traditional rule should be to add one or two more scoops or teaspoons of vinegar than vegetable oil. So, if for instance, you are making a salad for six, you will make a salad dressing with:

- 10 teaspoons of vegetable oil (olive oil preferably)

- 12 teaspoons of vinegar (notice the more spoons of vinegar added compared to the oil)

- Add a little bit of salt, black pepper, and herbs.

- You can also add one or two teaspoons of mayonnaise to make it tastier, but it's up to you.

- Shake or stir the mixture.

- Finish the process by adding it to your salad bowl or plate.

- Keep the remaining healthy salad dressing refrigerated. You can keep it for two to three weeks in the refrigerator.

BENEFITS: Preparing your own salads at home gives you control of what you put in them and also how much you put in. With this simple salad recipe, although you've added 10 teaspoons of vegetable oil, you will not consume it all in one day, but rather over a longer period because it's enough for several more salads in the days ahead. This is definitely a lighter alternative

TASK: Try making this salad recipe yourself and note how many calories are in 10 teaspoons of vegetable oil, 12 teaspoons of vinegar, and two teaspoons of mayonnaise.

Read the "Nutrition Facts" or Google these ingredients to find out, and then make a label for your salad dressing. Then, see how this compares with the number of calories in pre-made salads at the store. After that, move your pre-made salads (if you have any) to the left side of the fridge. Or if you were planning to buy some pre-made salads before attempting to make your own, cross them off your grocery list.

MISTAKE #3:
Not-So-Diet "Diet" Drinks

Just like with "low-fat" and "fat-free," don't let the word "diet" fool you. Yes, diet soda usually contains less sugar in it than regular soda, but that doesn't mean you are going to lose weight. And with the ongoing debate over the years about the safety of sugar substitutes like aspartame and saccharin, you may not want to put these things in your body anyway.

<u>REASONS</u>: Some doctors have linked diet soda to a number of health problems, including:

- High blood sugar;
- High blood pressure;

- Negatively impacting the bacteria in your gut, which is a diabetes risk;
- And some of these diet sodas may have more sugar in them than you think.

According to nutritionist Allison Sylvetsky Meni from the Milken Institute School of Public Health in Washington, D.C., people who consume diet soda are at higher risk of obesity than those who don't.

BENCHMARK: The best way to avoid this problem is to avoid diet soda and replace it with water or other healthier alternatives like homemade lemonade or iced tea.

BENEFITS: Water is healthier than any other drink and helps eliminate toxins, which can really facilitate your weight loss plan. When it comes to homemade drinks (lemonade or iced tea), you can control how much sugar you add, or none at all, to your mixture.

<u>TASK</u>: Learn to make your personal savory drinks by recreating all the traditional tasty beverages that your aunt or grandmother used to make. To make things simpler, when it comes to measuring the amount of sugar in your drink, treat it like a cup of coffee.

- Prepare your bottle of iced tea or lemonade without adding sugar.

- Every time you feel like having a glass, just add one, two or three teaspoons (not more) of sugar to your glass.

- Finish this task by moving all your diet sodas to the left of the fridge or pantry like the rest of the unhealthy/unwanted food.

MISTAKE #4:
"Low-Calorie" Condiments Trap

The word "calorie" has been thrown around countless times in the health and fitness industry to the point where now anything that is deemed as "low-calorie" is like the best thing since sliced bread (with sliced cheese and gravy).

Foods would be absolutely dull and completely unsatisfying without all the possible flavors they have to offer, and one of the simplest ways that we can custom tweak those flavors is through the different combination of condiments. To make us feel less guilty about enjoying too much of a good thing, manufacturers are pushing out these so-called "low-calorie" condiments so we can continue to overindulge.

Avoid this "low-calorie" trap, even if you are encouraged to still enjoy eating tasty meals while dieting. It's sad in some ways because you would think that with new technologies and new demands of the food market (where people want to eat healthier), we would have more legitimate options. But it's clearly not the case.

<u>REASONS</u>: Unfortunately, you still have to be careful with the advertising claims of low-calorie condiments like ketchup, mayonnaise, and salad dressings, etc. They are still loaded with sugar to make them taste good. Expert nutritionists like Ro Huntriss, the dietician behind the Terri-Ann-123 Diet Plan, see these low-calorie condiments as a big problem because of all the extra calories they add to your diet. Even if they end up having less sugar than your regular condiments, they still end up with unnecessary sugar, which is not good in the long run.

<u>BENCHMARK</u>: Once again, learn to make your own sauce for your vegetables, baked chicken, or rice. (You can refer to one recipe coming up for your task).

<u>BENEFITS</u>: You get to control and measure what you decide to eat as well as avoid potential risks of diabetes, high blood pressure, obesity, and other health issues related to too much sugar intake.

<u>TASK</u>: Substitute your low-calorie condiments with something self-made like your own dips and sauce with your low-fat meal. It's fairly simple and can be quite fun to experiment in the kitchen. Here, we will be making your own homemade tomato sauce with the following:

1. Put two fresh tomatoes with the stems removed in your blender and puree it.

2. Dice up some onions that you will fry for one minute (in two tablespoons of olive oil) together with minced garlic and some seasoning. Add a little bit of water to prevent your onions from burning.

3. Pour in your tomato puree into your pan with the onions and garlic.

4. Add salt for taste and stir until you get a consistent mix.

5. You can also add some pepper and herbs towards the end if desired.

6. Pour your tomato sauce over your favorite meal or dip it with your favorite side dish.

7. If there is any left, you can save it in the refrigerator for up to three days.

Now you can move all your low-fat condiments to the left side of your fridge or pantry.

MISTAKE #5:
Presumably Healthy Pescetarianism

Now let's talk about sushi. Huh, sushi? Yes, this may seem out of place, but sushi can be very deceiving for you fish lovers. On your plate it looks so fresh, lean, and natural. Besides, if you take a look at the Japanese society, a majority of Japanese people are already naturally slim through their everyday diet.

Then what is the problem? Well, as it turns out for you sushi fanatics hoping to satisfy your pescatarian hunger by eating all the sushi you can, that may be a bad idea.

<u>REASONS</u>: The sweet sauces and certain types of sushi like shrimp tempura rolls are very rich in calories. And if you like to enjoy your sushi every night as a "healthy meal," you should really take a closer look at what is on your platter. Some nutritionists like Ilyse Schapiro, a registered dietician and co-author of *Should I Scoop Out My Bagel?* even recommend substituting sushi for healthier alternatives like trout and salmon.

<u>BENCHMARK</u>: There is still a way to enjoy sushi when you are on a diet. Just make sure you skip sushi that is filled with too much sauce or fried seafood. Instead, go for rolls with fresh vegetables, avocado, fresh or grilled fish, and also opt for the ones with brown rice rather than white rice because brown rice has more fiber and nutrients on top being linked to weight loss.

<u>BENEFITS</u>: You can eat healthier sushi as much as you want without worrying about putting on weight because fresh vegetables are processed much faster into your system, and healthy sushi has more nutrients than the ones that are

saturated with rich sauces just to make them more appealing.

TASK: If you love sushi and eat it regularly, broaden your list of options when it comes to sushi by making a restricted list, so you will eat only healthy sushi with fresh fish and vegetables and also with brown rice instead of white.

MISTAKE #6:
The Overhyped Upgrade to Water

Ah, coconut water has become the miracle drink for many dieters and those who seek a healthier life because of its health benefits. Some people believe it has antioxidant properties, making it great for those with diabetes, and that it may reduce blood pressure. It is also a delicious tropical drink. But you have to be careful about how much coconut water you actually consume.

REASONS: Well, according to Lilian Cheung, director of health promotion and communication at the Harvard School of Public Health's Department of Nutrition, coconut water contains a lot of sugar. For example, for every one cup of coconut water, you will ingest 45 calories and six grams of sugar. So, if you drink eight cups of coconut water per day, you consume 48 grams of sugar. That's a lot! In the long run, your weight loss efforts will be destined to fail because you are consuming more sugar than you should.

BENCHMARK: Find yourself a healthy drink with similar qualities but less sugar and fewer calories. Green tea is a great option. And remember, you can always just drink good old water.

BENEFITS: Green tea is traditionally known to help with weight loss (although no modern study can attest to that), and it contains much fewer calories than coconut water (one cup contains only 1 calorie). Water (distilled or purified) will help you get rid of toxins, which can help you lose weight more effectively.

TASK: It may prove arduous giving up on your love of coconut water but try to move all your containers of coconut water to the left side of your fridge or pantry and replace them with water or green tea on the right side. Compare your weight before and after abstaining from your coco-nutty friend. That should be motivating enough for you for the long term.

MISTAKE #7:
Unmoderated Breakfast Cereals

For many people, cereal has been part of their morning routine since childhood and promotes a feeling of home comfort. We have always considered cereal to be a healthy and helpful breakfast, especially for kids, because it usually contains fiber, and there are so many varieties and flavors available. But, watch out!

According to nutritionist Hrefna Palsdottir, although cereals are delicious and very convenient, they too should be eaten carefully when you want to lose weight. And this isn't just about the obviously sugary cereals that appeal to children. This includes what we normally think of as healthy cereals, such as "Grape Nuts," for example.

<u>REASONS</u>: There are many different varieties of cereals, each with their flavorful appeal. They sometimes have too many calories in such a small unexpected quantity. For instance, for one bowl of Grape Nuts cereal has about 416 calories with 590 milligrams of sodium (salt). The other problem is that you don't eat cereal alone. By adding milk, you are putting more calories and fat into your bowl. Instead of losing weight you are either stagnating or putting on weight over time. At the end of the day, cereal is essentially another colorful-packaged product to get you to come back for more; otherwise, you might as well eat plain grains that are boring in taste.

<u>BENCHMARK</u>: You should minimize your cereal intake by maybe replacing it with a bowl of fresh fruit, or scrambled eggs for breakfast during the week. It's all about portions here. And make sure to use low-fat milk with your cereal to help minimize the long-term fattening effect it may have on you.

<u>BENEFITS</u>: You get more nutrients in fruits but also more fiber and less fat and sugar.

<u>TASK</u>: Revise your weekly eating plan by eating more fruits for breakfast (which should replace some of the meals that included a bowl of cereal during the week). If you were eating cereal four times a week because you felt it gave you energy and more fiber to help with digestion, reduce it to one bowl of cereal during the week, and the rest of the week you can alternate with either boiled or scrambled eggs, or fruit (a variety of fruit like bananas, strawberries, oranges, apples, etc.). Make sure you eat at least three to five servings of fruit in the morning and try to balance that intake (so that you don't end up bloated) by eating one big fruit (like oranges, bananas, apples, etc.) against a variety of four little fruits (strawberries, grapes, berries, etc.). You can still eat cereal, but with moderation.

MISTAKE #8:
Too Much of an Oily Good Thing

Many people who choose to eat healthier prefer olive oil. It is said to be more natural and polyvalent (because you can use it on your skin or your hair and benefit from its soothing and nourishing qualities). But before you start pouring on the olive oil, there's something you should know.

It turns out that olive oil is not the best thing in the world for your weight if you don't control how much is actually in your food. You don't have to cut olive oil from your diet entirely, but you should reduce how much you consume.

<u>REASONS</u>: It is important to know how rich this oil is and how bad it could be for your weight if you consume too much. Even though you might not feel or see the effects right away, you should keep in mind that 1/4 cup of olive oil alone has almost 500 calories and over 50 grams of fat! For those who cook regularly and use measuring cups, you know that 1/4 cup is a very small quantity. And 500 calories is huge for such a small ingredient.

<u>BENCHMARK</u>: Limit your olive oil intake by making boiled vegetables instead of sautéed vegetables. Use a teaspoon to measure the quantity of olive oil you use when you want to fry or sauté your meat. If you are in the habit of pouring olive oil everywhere, stop immediately, or at least limit it to no more than one teaspoon per dish.

<u>BENEFITS</u>: By using only one teaspoon, the oil is processed through your body more easily, and its nutrients are absorbed without retaining any fats. So, it's almost as if you weren't consuming any oil in the end because you'll now be using only what you truly need.

TASK: From now on, go for these cooking alternatives to diminish and control how much olive oil you use in your diet:

- Use the one teaspoon rule, where you will strictly use only one teaspoon of olive oil in your dishes.

- Favor boiling over frying when it comes to vegetables.

The olive oil can stay in your cabinet (keeping it on your right side) as it is still a healthy alternative to vegetable oil.

MISTAKE #9:
Bottled Health Beverages

The popular belief is that since there are so many "weight-loss-friendly" health foods and beverages out there, it means you can consume as much of them as you want. *Don't be fooled by such feel-good crap!*

Green tea is believed to help with weight loss. The same can be said about green smoothies; when it comes to smoothies, they are just a liquified version of your four to five vegetables or fruits a day (and the fact that you blend them makes it easier to ingest them at once). So, overall, they all seem to be healthy and safe options for dieters.

The problem is, the food industry adds things to these drinks to make them more appealing to consumers. (Let's face it, drinking plain green smoothies can sometimes intolerably taste like grass.) As a result, the consumer version of these products is not as healthy as advertised, according to Dan Nadeau, medical director of Exeter Hospital's Health Reach Diabetes, Endocrinology and Nutrition Center in New Hampshire.

<u>REASONS</u>: The truth is that these bottled health drinks might not give you the benefits that you are looking for or be more effective than regular sodas because they are generally mixed with other types of diluters. This, in turn, decreases their potency and adds more sugar to your diet. When it comes to bottled smoothies, numbers don't lie. Some smoothies can have between 600 and 1,000 calories in a single bottle and are loaded with sugar!

<u>BENCHMARK</u>: You should make your own healthy drinks at home by simply putting a few green tea bags into a pitcher of water and storing them in your fridge. Buy the

whole vegetables and fruits to be blended into your homemade power smoothies.

BENEFITS: You definitely reduce your sugar intake here and you are also absorbing more nutrients that will help you cleanse your body and carry on with your weight loss program.

TASK: As a mini task, prepare one or two bottles of tea (boil two bags of green tea per bottle) and keep them on the right side of your fridge. Move any store-bought bottled health drinks to the left side of your fridge because eventually you will want them completely cleansed from your fridge for good.

MISTAKE #10:
Fake Fruit Juices

Many people drink canned or bottled fruit juices instead of eating actual fruit because they assume drinking a glass of juice is the equivalent of eating a few servings of fruit per day. If you believe that and you are trying to lose weight, then you'll be in for a big surprise.

<u>REASONS</u>: During the production process, fruit juices lose all their fiber consistency, which you need to help digest your food, especially now that you are trying to eat healthier and lose weight. In other words, they are totally empty in fiber (even for 100% fruit juices), according to nutrition expert Dan Nadeau, whom we mentioned earlier. So, these fruit concentrate juices hardly have any real

nutritional value and are usually full of added sugar, like drinking Kool-Aid.

BENCHMARK: Avoid the standard store-shelved fruit juices and preferably make your own natural fruit juices at home. Here's how:

- Peel and wash all fruits before juicing them because juice tastes better without the rough, starchy feeling of the peels.

- Add two large fruits (such as oranges and apples, peeled and chopped). For even bigger fruits like pineapple or watermelon, chop them and add two bowls full. For smaller fruits, (strawberries, blueberries, grapes, etc.) just add one bowl full.

- Get out your juicer.

- You don't need to add water at all.

- Don't forget to store your homemade juices in the fridge and drink them as much as you can because naturally-made products don't last as long unless you freeze them (a minor con that is being outweighed by the major pro of having real healthier fruit juices served).

<u>BENEFITS</u>: You preserve all necessary fibers (your gut will thank you for that). You have fewer chances of getting constipated during your diet, and you also preserve all the nutrients needed by your body. Remember that one of the golden rules of dieting is not to cut off any nutrients because your body still needs them. When it comes to water, you should already know the benefits, which is to help you eliminate toxins that can be harmful to your body.

<u>TASK</u>: Try juicing five or six fruits at home using our rule:

- 2 big peeled fruits (oranges or apples)
- 2 bowls of super big fruits (pineapple or watermelon)
- 1 bowl of smaller fruits (strawberries or blueberries)

- Add and juice them progressively in the juicer.

- Makes one serving (approximately 200 to 300 milliliters)

- No sugar or water is needed.

End the process by moving all the fruit juices from your local grocery store's shelf aisle to the left side of your fridge as a reminder to avoid them from now on.

MISTAKE #11:
The Everyday Beloved Superfood

Next on our list is a little shocker, because it is none other than the "avocado." People love avocadoes, and they are considered to be superfoods and are desirable as an everyday salad topper or food dip and spread.

Although it is a healthy fruit, when you overeat avocadoes you might end up packing on some unexpected weight. The worst part, you won't ever suspect that it comes from this type of food (so you probably will be taken aback when eating healthy "by the book," yet your clothes start to feel a little tighter than usual...and you've never even washed them!)

<u>REASONS</u>: Well, avocados turn out to be fattening in the long run when you don't control your portions because the average one has about 300 calories. Nutritionists like Taylor Jones agree that they are a great source of vitamins and minerals, but, unfortunately, they are high in fat. If you enjoy cutting up an avocado and adding it to your favorite salads during the week, this could mean that you are ingesting the equivalent of two ice cream sandwiches! Even though avocadoes have some monounsaturated fats that are good for you, you should diminish your portions during the week.

<u>BENCHMARK</u>: Try eating half of an avocado instead of a whole one. Or try other salad toppers that are less fattening, such as:

- Chopped pieces of an apple, which add a sweet touch to your salads, have plenty of minerals and are traditionally known to help fight obesity. An average size apple only has 95 calories and less than a half a gram of fat.

- One tablespoon of sliced almonds which contains protein and healthy fats. One tablespoon only has 40 calories and three-and-a-half grams of fat.

<u>BENEFITS</u>: This way you still absorb a variety of nutrients but with less fat than if you were using only avocados to top your salads during the week.

<u>TASK</u>: Try reducing your avocado consumption by adding other healthier alternatives like apples, sliced almonds, etc. Do your research to make sure that whatever you substitute to your salad has less fat and fewer calories than an avocado. From now on, only eat avocados once a week. You can still keep your avocados, but just make sure you eat them in smaller quantities.

MISTAKE #12:
The Case of "Unhealthy Vegetables"

Vegetables being associated with the word "unhealthy" might come as a surprise to many. After all, vegetables have always been thought of as the healthiest things out there. Although your veggies can be a great source of nutrients as well as a great source of energy, not all of them should be consumed when dieting.

"Starchy" vegetables like corn and potatoes have been proven to lead to weight gain for people who constantly add them to their diets.

<u>REASONS</u>: Potatoes, for instance, have been proven to be effective only for short-term weight loss. But in the long run, they can slow your metabolism and also decrease muscle mass. Corn is no different and is also considered bad for weight loss because it can potentially cause you to add two pounds of weight for every additional serving over four years, according to Eric Rimm, professor of medicine at the Harvard Medical School.

<u>BENCHMARK</u>: Professor Rimm recommends replacing these two starchy vegetables with high fiber green vegetables like kale and string beans for better weight loss results.

<u>BENEFITS</u>: Kale and string beans are both rich in antioxidants and nutrients like vitamin C and collagen (which you do need while dieting) and are also easily broken down by your digestive system.

<u>TASK</u>: Try erasing the "starchy" vegetables like potatoes and corn from your grocery list and only focus on eating

green vegetables that can speed up your weight loss plan or cause fewer problems. If you already have string beans and kale on your list, buy twice as much as you usually do so you will eat more.

MISTAKE #13:
The Forbidden Fruits when Dieting

Just like with the vegetables we mentioned prior, there are also some fruits that you should avoid if you want to lose weight. For example, another "starchy" sinner is banana. Did you know that one banana can have more carbs than two slices of white bread? You should also watch out for dried fruits because they are also very starchy.

<u>REASONS</u>: Alissa Rumsey, nutrition therapist and certified intuitive eating counselor, cautions that a medium-sized banana has about 27 grams of carbs and 14 grams of sugar. That's quite a bit more than two slices of white bread. As for dried fruits, Anthony Komaroff,

executive editor of the Harvard Health Letter, says that because dried fruits are so small, we tend to eat too many. The big problem is that some food producers add sugar to dried fruits. Even just one ounce of certain dried fruits may contain 120 calories.

BENCHMARK: Alissa Rumsey recommends not completely getting rid of your bananas but changing the way you eat them. It's okay to eat them right before or after your workout sessions because bananas can help fuel your workout and recovery. When it comes to packaged dried fruits, try to stay away from them as much as you can because you never know how much sugar you are truly ingesting. Stick to more natural sources of sugar like apples, oranges, and grapes.

BENEFITS: Using bananas for more functional reasons in your diet plan (like recovery and refueling) effectively lowers their consumption, thus preventing you from putting on too much unnecessary weight. Also, eliminating dried fruits will help you decrease more risks of adding unnecessary sugar to your diet.

<u>TASK</u>: You can keep your bananas for your workout sessions, but move your dried fruits to the left side of the fridge or pantry and don't bother restocking them now that you know why.

MISTAKE #14:
The Bloody Red Meat

While animal protein is the densest one when it comes to nutrients (it is especially rich in iron), you still have to be mindful of your meat choices. Although red meat like beef, for instance, possesses a high amount of protein, it is really not a healthy alternative when it comes to getting your dose of animal protein while dieting (because remember, you need all your nutrients even when trying to lose weight).

REASONS: Let's look at the numbers. In a three-ounce serving of lean beef, you will consume 180 calories, according to Shalene McNeill with the National Cattlemen's Beef Association. That's huge compared to a three-ounce serving of white meat (like lean chicken) where you'll get 140 calories. And a three-ounce serving of Atlantic cod has only around 90 calories.

<u>BENCHMARK</u>: Eat less red meat and go for chicken, turkey, and fish. If you are still confused about when you should eat red meat, try eating it only once a month. This way you maximize your consumption of healthy meats (white meats) and you even reduce the risks of diseases that you may get by eating too much red meat.

<u>BENEFITS</u>: You minimize your consumption in saturated fats that can increase your cholesterol and also reduce your consumption of unnecessary fats that could ruin your diet in the long run. Also, remember that your decision to go on a diet is not only to have a healthy weight but also to avoid certain health problems later down the road that may occur when you consume too much animal fat (like high cholesterol and heart disease).

<u>TASK</u>: Find ways to add variety in how you cook your fish and chicken so you have more alternatives to eating red meat.

MISTAKE #15:
A Nutty Glutton

In general, nuts are known to be good sources of fat, fiber, and protein. Most of their fat is monounsaturated fat, and Omega 6 and 3 polyunsaturated fats. However, when dieting you need to eat nuts in moderation. Nuts are small, so we tend to eat too many of them. A half-ounce of nuts like cashews and pistachios could contain 15 grams of fat!

<u>REASONS</u>: It is obviously because nuts are high in fat and calories. For most nuts like Brazil nuts and cashews, one serving contains around 160 calories or more. Eating more calories than your body burns, in the long run, could lead to weight gain.

<u>BENCHMARK</u>: Try storing your nuts in small containers:

- Use a small container which should be half as small as a cereal bowl and consider it your serving of nuts for the whole day.

- Pace yourself only eating nuts twice a week as an afternoon snack. This way you can feel fuller sooner by not gulping them down hastily, minimize your cravings, and also get enough polyunsaturated and monounsaturated fats.

<u>BENEFITS</u>: You get to effectively balance your consumption of "healthy fats" without depriving yourself of the benefits they can bring to your body and to your health during your dieting.

<u>TASK</u>: Add a tiny bowl or container to your list of daily utensils in order to help you measure your portions of nuts twice a week for your afternoon snack. You can keep your nuts on the right side of your cabinet or pantry, as long as

you follow the portioning method so you will not consume too much fat at once.

ENCORE ACT:
Tasks to Follow Suit

<u>TASK 1</u>: Reduce overconsumption using portion methods or bring more variety to your meals:

1. Pick vegetables that you normally eat every week.

2. Research how many calories each one of them has.

3. For those with more than 100 calories, reduce your consumption to once every seven days (once per week).

4. For the rest, you can still eat them regularly, as your body will have less trouble breaking them down during the digestion phase.

TASK 2: Get used to using less oil—like olive oil—by reducing it to one teaspoon for your meals, while still getting the benefits of it.

- For salad, sprinkle one teaspoon.

- For vegetable, stir it frequently while sautéing.

- For meat, use a fork to poke small holes to cook the meat more evenly, as cooking meat with little oil can make the meat look dry/burn or cook faster only on the outside. (Remember, meat is ideal for protein but should be eaten moderately when dieting.)

TASK 3: Another way to reduce your olive oil consumption is to alternate with coconut oil, which is similar in calorie and fat content. Coconut oil is said to help reduce belly fat. The daily recommendation is two tablespoons (30 milliliters) a day. What you should do is alternate by using:

- Coconut oil for baking and frying (using two tablespoons).

- Olive oil for your salads from now on (using one teaspoon).

TASK 4: Finish the fridge and pantry organizing session by getting rid of all the items that are too fattening to eat during your weight loss program. You can donate these items to a food shelter or give them to someone who is not trying to lose weight. Now then, box everything up and give it to someone in need.

F(ULL) ACE AT REVEAL:
Knowingly Demystified Healthy Foods

Losing weight can be a surprisingly exciting experience because it's no longer a one-trip pony where you need to do some specific complicated yo-yo exercising and can only lose weight fast (by restricting yourself to starving) and wind up gaining it all back. Instead, there are many diverse ways of going about it.

Nowadays, dieting is just a matter of willpower and not that much of a constraint anymore because you can find exactly what you need at the grocery store. The real problem is the many deceptive "low-fat" and "healthy" meals being advertised as ideal for weight loss, but they are packed with loads of sugar, fat, and added hidden ingredients that can easily sabotage your diet.

The best way to avoid this problem is to understand as much as possible about what is really in the food you are eating, especially those tricky items that you think are healthy but in reality are not. Keep a list of these misleading foods with you and hang it on your fridge as a reminder of how easy it is to make mistakes when you are trying to decide what to eat.

With all the information that you know have at your disposal, enjoy your weight loss program and say bye-bye to the weight for good and keep it that way by maintaining your healthy diet always.

www.ingramcontent.com/pod-product-compliance
Lightning Source LLC
Chambersburg PA
CBHW050655250726

48662CB00002B/690